Twelve Weeks to Fertility

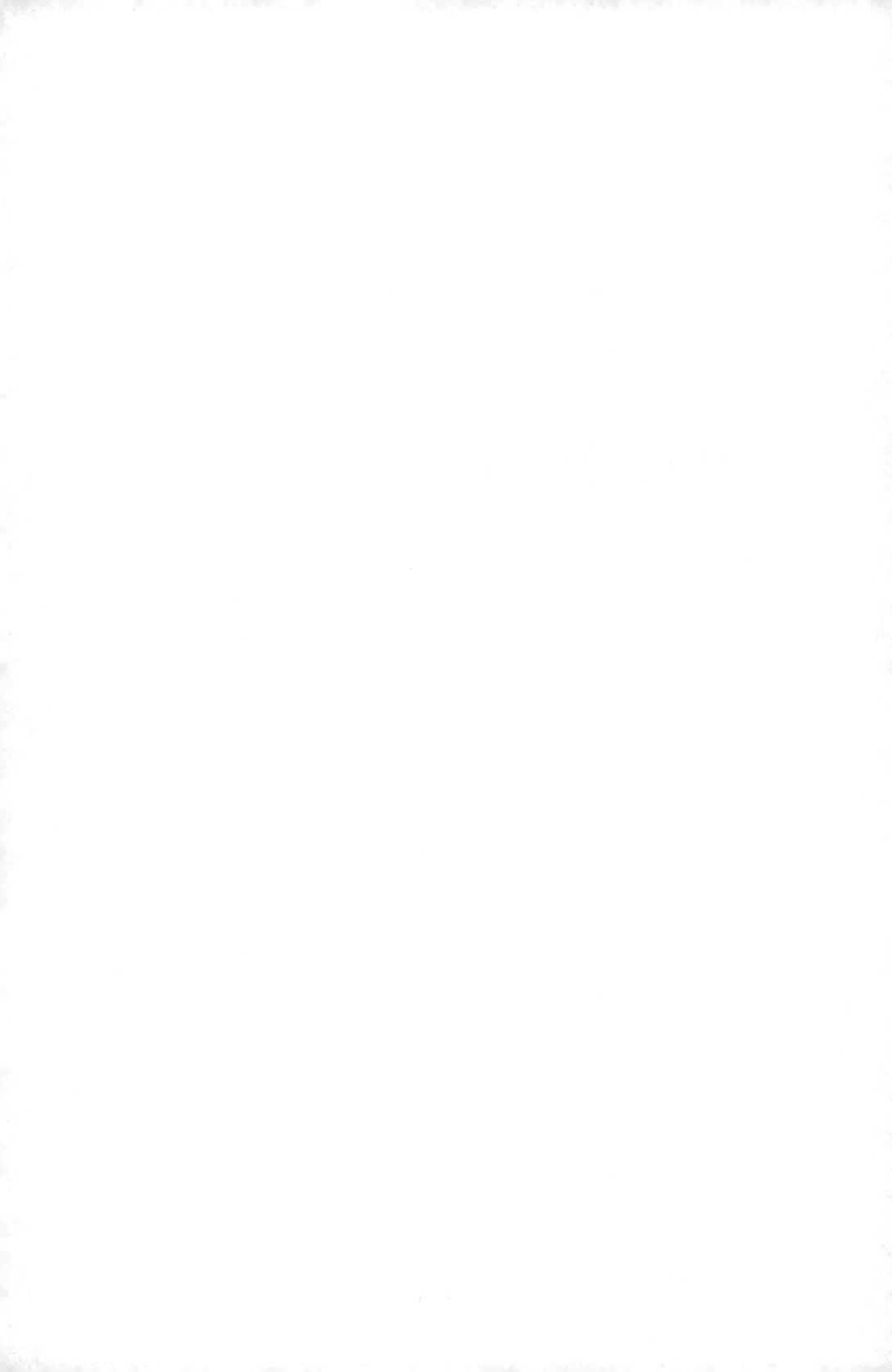

Twelve Weeks to Fertility

The Easy Way to Conceive and Carry a
Healthy Baby to Full Term

Michelle Leclaire O'Neill, Ph.D., R.N.

Writers Club Press
San Jose New York Lincoln Shanghai

Twelve Weeks to Fertility
The Easy Way to Conceive and to Carry a Healthy Baby to Full Term

Writers Club Press
an imprint of iUniverse.com, Inc.

For information address:
iUniverse.com, Inc.
5220 S 16th, Ste. 200
Lincoln, NE 68512
www.iuniverse.com

ISBN: 0-595-14841-7

Printed in the United States of America

This book is dedicated to all the fertility mothers and fathers that I have had the privilege of working with.

Your journeys are amazing. This truly is a new and different and very exciting evolutionary time.

And

With deep appreciation to O. Carl Simonton, M.D. for his pioneering work in Mind/Body Medicine

Thou camst upon things dying
And I upon things newborn
William Shakespeare

Contents

Preface

How to use this Book in the most time efficient way for body/mind success:

Weeks 1–8—Read one chapter a week (you may read chapter 8 & 9 together). You do not have to do any of the exercises in the chapters until you have read the entire book.

Week 9—Now that you are finished reading you may do the exercises in chapter 6.

Week 10—You may now do exercises in chapter 4.

Week 11—You are now ready to do the exercise in chapter 2.

Week 12—Write out your 12-week health plan in chapter 9. Make four copies—give one to your partner, put one on the bathroom mirror, one in the kitchen and keep one with you. Review plan once a week for 5 minutes with your partner. I will listen to your progress and/or difficulty with health plan and I would like you to listen to my progress and/or difficulty. Set a definite time e.g. every Wednesday from 8–8:15 p.m.

You may now begin to write in your Fertility Journal at the back of the book.

All the exercises are for both parents to be.

If you think you are doing this alone; there are many other mothers who are doing this alone. Try to find a way to connect to each other.

Put a notice on your Doctors Bulletin Board. Start a group on the Internet. Start a local Fertility 12-week group using this book as a guide. Contact me for groups in your area, or post your group on my website @ *www.hypnobirthing.ws*, email *Birthing@gte.net* (please leave your phone number whenever you email)

Chapter One

Elemental Rhythms:
The Evolution of the Leclaire Fertility Method

While my father was on his way to Europe to fight in World War II, I was born at the Harkness Pavilion of Columbia-Presbyterian Hospital in New York City into an Italian, Catholic household, in an Irish parish. Here, early feelings, emotions, rules and routines were imprinted on my body, mind and soul.

In the beginning, the days in the neighborhood were soft and time-less. There were many gentle men in my life. Best among them was my Grandpapa, Salvatore, who knew about life. He had the luck of the Irish—it happens sometimes to Italians. At the age of two, when he first arrived in New York, he fell out of a third-story window and safely rolled onto the awning below. He knew about rhythms. It was he who told my mother how to care for me, as she deliberated on which book of male wisdom to follow in feeding me. His advice was, "When she's hungry, she'll cry—feed her then. When she's tired, she'll sleep—let her. When she's sad, she'll have another cry—console her. It's as simple as that. Throw out the clock, she's too young to tell time."

He remained "too young to tell time" all his life, which meant he had time for everything. He went to mass and communion every morning, played the horses every afternoon, listened to opera every evening as he cooked for us all, took me anywhere I wanted to go and let me be whoever I was at the moment. We had a great friendship, an inter-generational love affair that has lasted all my life.

But when the war was over and the men came home, my soft, rhythmical world became one of order and rules. The women stopped driving trucks and working in factories and the soul-burned men took over. They slept on floors—beds, apparently, were not enough like fox holes. They lived by clocks and watches. They made contracts, which they broke whenever they remembered or heard in their minds the distant sound of bombs bursting in air. They were here—but they were still there—and their rules replaced their rhythms. They felt safe with rules, and each time their fear returned, they would make harder rules and more stringent laws. So it was that the men lost their melody and forced those who lived by life's natural rhythms to abide by what they thought was right and reasonable.

As this rhythmical world disappeared, the children began to get sick. They were paralyzed and they needed iron lungs to breathe. They could no longer walk in the tall grass and smell the fragrance of the lilacs in spring or go sledding on the empty hills in winter, dodging trees and rocks with ease. They were frozen in their paths. The great germ of the war had come home to infect the children. If they didn't have polio, they were paralyzed in another way—emotionally. They had to sit on the stoop. They couldn't swim, they couldn't play with the children across the street for fear of contracting germs. With a shadow over them, they had to nap from noon to three each afternoon. Everyday like Good Friday. Those children who survived grew up to meet and deal with other epidemics—of cancer, aids and infertility. Did the sickness come to bring them back to their own flow, to their own way of being? Did the sickness come out of the darkness to bring light again and flowering time? We don't know but, through all this, the real people like my Grandpapa continued to live by their own elemental rhythms, by the light and the shadow of the sun. I've learned that it is from that light and through that shadow that the healing power of life is found.

Recently I was very much involved with two patients in their thirties—a woman with recurrent breast cancer on the cusp of death and a woman trying to get pregnant after two abortions and one miscarriage. One not ready to die and another not quite ready to conceive. Neither seemed able to grasp what she had to do to move toward life and the life force. Yet -at the deepest level—each knew what she needed to do. All of us know, but it is often easier to hide from that knowledge than it is to be or to act.

Fertility is not only found in the daily injections of ovarian hormonal stimulation's or in lab fertilized embryos. It is not only in blood tests and ultrasounds which witness the progressive growth of the uterine lining. It is not in the many years and thousands of dollars spent on insemination, surgery and in-vitro fertilization. Somewhere between the light and the shadow of the sun and the gentle breeze of the sea, somewhere in the balance of our mind, body, and spirit, the return to healing and fertility takes place.

The Leclaire Fertility Method described in this book works on the level of needed repair, which neither drugs nor surgery nor even acupuncture nor herbs can touch. It will help you to create a climate in which healing can take place, so that you can give nature a chance to move freely within. Only you have the power to reawaken this innate intelligence and to restore balance and health to your life.

Drs. Alan Beer and Joanne Kwak from the Department of Reproductive Medicine at the University of Chicago Medical School believe that "every pregnancy interacts with the maternal immune system." Leclaire is the study of that interaction—and of the communication which takes place among the psyche, the nervous system, the immune system, the endocrine system, and the reproductive system.

Disease has two manifestations:
1. Psychological and Spiritual
2. Physical and Biological

Our body is influenced by our surroundings, including,

the air we breathe,

the person who is our partner,

the friends with whom we socialize,

the literature we read,

the music we listen to,

the TV and films we watch,

the food we eat, and

the thoughts we think.

Therefore, all the elements of our lives have the potential to be medicine.

Many people try to feel better by attending to their material needs -for example, they buy a new car or suit or dress or a new set of golf clubs, or they have a face lift or a tummy tuck. There is nothing wrong with developing this part of your persona, but it is also important, while attending to your more superficial desires, not to deny your true self and their deep inner needs.

In our society it is hard not to buy into the belief that a certain kind of body—a very slender one—is perfect. That image is accepted and loved by the culture to which we want to belong. Having a body different from this model of perfection—which few of us can attain—means that we are excluded. Rather than having major surgery in order to belong, or becoming anorexic or bulimic, it would be healthier and much more gratifying to explore the reasons for feeling excluded, the origin of that feeling, as well as where you really want to belong. It may be that the society of perfect bodies represents for you acceptance by your mother. But, if it is impossible to gain acceptance from your mother, you could find social support in another group. I've seen this happen with several of my clients. One woman had a great need for approval, which she did not get from her family. She was blessed with an ability to write poetry so she started a poetry writing and reading group. She made that her new family of approval. Another woman decided to take singing lessons and then had recitals for small groups of friends who would support rather than judge her. Yet another woman started a feminist ecumenical group, where the women discussed the ways they felt they couldn't be themselves if they wanted acceptance in their churches, their synagogues, their families and their neighborhoods. Good things happen to people who are in tune with their elemental rhythms, and who are willing to seek the inner truth.

Emotions are the road signs on the journey which each of us must choose for ourselves. We must follow those signposts. If we do not, the same emotion will come up again and again and again—until we deal with it, or until it deals with us through progressive symptoms and disease. It is sometimes necessary for us to get sick before we will listen to the self trying to emerge. We do not behave this way because we want to be sick or self destructive. We behave the way we do because it is easier than attempting to change. We love and are comfortable with the familiar, even if the familiar hurts. If, however, we have the tools and support for change, and if we can deal with our fear of change, we can each move in the direction of new and healthier beliefs and behaviors.

Physicians are trained to gather all of the symptoms and information relevant to their patient's condition and then to develop a diagnosis and a treatment plan. What they are not taught—and what they therefore often leave out—is the meaning behind the symptoms, the spirit or true cause of the illness.

Science, like medicine, operates in the realm of objective fact, but many of the issues surrounding fertility are in the domain of subjective values. It is within this domain that we will explore the path from infertility to fertility in this book. In today's society, infertility may not be entirely due to the individual couple's problems. It may also be a social problem, one related to our culture's priorities. It may, in part, stem from our current technology, which is in many ways destructive to both our environment and the intuitive/maternal way of thinking. It is my intent in this book to have you join me in discovering and walking a path which will preserve the delicate balance between male and female, between technology and Mother Earth, between facts and values, between rational and intuitive thought, between reproductive medicine and mind/body healing.

During the course of this book you will learn easy ways to make changes which will help you achieve your goals and allow you to be happier, more relaxed and more content. You will be taught how to reach physiological, emotional and spiritual balance with minimal effort. If you use the techniques of this program, it will be the gateway to rebuilding your mind/body/fertility bond and optimal state of health. It is all too easy—when you're trying so hard to attain a goal—to turn that path into a battle to be won. Instead, I see that quest as a silence to be heard, a path to be walked, a rhythm that flows, a moment to be lived now, in its own time, in the full presence of all that you can bring to it today. Please join me in an exploration and explanation of a different way of thinking and being.

Chapter Two

Claire's Story and Treatment

Before we begin the steps to fertility ourselves, let's look for a moment at Claire, a patient of mine who, like many of you reading this book, had difficulty conceiving. She had been a career woman for many years, doing well as a competitive swimmer and coach. She and her husband, Josh, ten years her junior, had one child, Timmy, now five years old. His conception was easy and uneventful and Claire enjoyed a normal pregnancy. After his birth, she became a full-time mother, a role she liked. She didn't miss her swimming and coaching activities. She took up painting and, between her artwork and her responsibilities as a mom and homemaker, she had neither the time nor the desire to work outside of her home.

Josh felt different. He wanted Claire to conceive, not only because they both wanted another child, but because he had gotten her to agree that once she was pregnant, she would go back to work. Claire was tremendously reluctant to return to work, although she never acknowledged this to Josh or anyone else.

When her son Timmy was two-and-a-half, Claire conceived and shortly thereafter had a miscarriage. She was devastated. When she was referred to me, she was still very depressed over this loss. She was losing weight, suffering from insomnia, migraine headaches and severe knee pain, for which she was using various pain medications. After exploring her feelings, she discovered that she was furious with Josh for insisting that she return to work as soon as she conceived.

She felt that they did not need the money and that his demands were acting as a deterrent both to conceiving and carrying a healthy baby to term. She realized that she no longer wanted to work outside of her home—she had done that for years. She now wanted to be a mother and homemaker. She wanted Josh to accept that role as an integral and important a part of maintaining the family—as important as his work in the business world.

Once Claire was able to admit this to herself, and to discuss it with Josh, he was willing to do a "Rational Thought Process" (which we will explore in depth later) to change his belief that motherhood is just "a cushy job." When he realized that his convictions were playing an important part in Claire's unconscious desire not to get pregnant, he was able to let go of his resentment about her staying home and change his pressuring behavior.

After dealing with these feelings, Claire was gradually able to give up her pain medication. Slowly she stopped having migraine headaches and knee pain.

Claire then followed the entire program—all the steps to fertility which are discussed in the chapters of this book. She incorporated meditation into her life. She then employed imagery and hypnosis first to relieve her pain, then to relax and visualize her life as she wanted it to be. Through working with her dreams, she was able to develop her own ideas, talents, attitudes and feelings, rather than blindly accepting those held dear by Josh. For years she had felt dominated and victimized by her in-laws. Now, using these same techniques, she was able to gain emotional mastery and alter her relationship with them.

One of the most important things Claire realized in taking these steps was that she had a pleasure freeze in her life. Sex had become only a way of conceiving. She also felt guilty and in conflict over many other areas of her life. This all began to change. Now, when Claire schedules a play date for her son, she often invites the child's mother so that she, too, can have some fun. At other times, she takes a few of Timmy's friends with her to the park and plays with them. She started swimming again—not competitively, not even timing herself or counting her laps—but for fun and as a part of her exercise program.

After Claire and Josh each did Step 1, a Rational Thought Process (RTP), Claire took all of the steps of the program as part of her 12 week health plan, which changed her outlook and entire way of living. Here are the goals she set for herself:

Play—Timmy and I will have a play date three times a week. On two of those dates, I will take Timmy and his friends on an outing which will be fun for us all. For example, we'll go to the YMCA pool and play water games.

Exercise—I will swim three times a week using a pull buoy so that I don't put more wear and tear on my knees.

Social Support—Even though Josh doesn't practice his religion, I want to go to my church on Sunday and participate in women's events at church twice a week.

Nutrition—I will not eat on the run. I will sit down while I eat and will rest for ten minutes after eating.

Creative Healing—My current goal is to get in touch with my creativity by taking time to paint and draw three times a week.

In addition to making the above commitments to herself, Claire worked the other steps of the program as follows:

a) *Meditation*—Initially, Claire found it difficult to sit still, but she began to learn meditation during our weekly sessions. At the beginning, she could only quiet her mind for five minutes at a time. Now, she is able to meditate for twenty minutes, five times a week.

b) *Hypnosis and Imagery*—Each week Claire participated in an hypnotic relaxation and concentration session, during which she became almost totally unaware of what was going on around her. She was, however, intensely conscious of a narrow range of stimuli which were called to her attention, and of the ideas which were suggested to her. Once, when she was under hypnosis, we went back into her childhood looking for times when she was truly happy. At one point she began to cry, realizing how intimate she had been with her friends in high school and how she longed for such intimacy in her life today.

We then employed imagery, which utilizes the senses as a means of realizing goals. As we'll see more examples of throughout this book, imagery can actually affect emotional perceptions and even create bodily changes. Claire used her imagination to create the life she wanted. She visualized herself pain free, in a certain community, living in a house they owned rather than the rented home in which they lived. She saw herself holding a baby girl -Rosemarie—in her arms. While Timmy and his friends played and jumped about, Claire was engaged in a conversation with three other young mothers. She was anticipating Josh's return home from work that evening with particular excitement because they were invited for dinner at a friend's house with three other couples.

c) *Dreams*—Claire recorded her dreams and her emotions, specifically those which made her angry. She found that her dreams and her anger were related. It was through this step that she began to feel safe and confident enough to alter her relationship with her in-laws and to let go of feeling trapped and isolated.

d) *Therapeutic touch and/or acupuncture*—Claire had 15 weekly acupuncture treatments. Acupuncture can normalize and restore the optimum condition of the reproductive organs for fertility.

Claire measured her overall success through increased happiness, moments of joy and serenity, self-acceptance, better sleep, the disappearance of her migraine headaches and knee pain, increased social support, letting go of her addiction to pain medication and better communication with Josh. She believes that both her attitudes and her biochemistry have undergone quite a transformation, making her ready to conceive and to carry a healthy baby to full term.

Chapter Three

The Rational Thought Process

You are most likely reading this book now because of your desire to have a child. This is a unique life situation, which this book specifically addresses. The material in this and other chapters, however, is also designed to help you cope better with absolutely anything. You will learn clear-cut methods for dealing with self-defeating emotions which may be inhibiting you. The first step towards fertility is to move in the direction of achieving personal happiness and this chapter provides a plan to help you do that.

To benefit from this book, you must invest some time. If you do, you will be thrilled and amazed at how the simple techniques presented here can lead to permanent personal happiness.

We all act on our thoughts. What we feel and do is a result of our thinking. If you are like most people, some of your thinking is healthy and some is unhealthy. Our thoughts and ideas have come from our parents, families, schools, the media, our churches, temples, organizations, social support groups and physicians. Before any idea or thought can influence our emotional feelings or our physical action, however, we have to think it, believe it and then react to it. As fallible human beings, we normally react to both healthy and unhealthy beliefs. This chapter is about learning how to take the unhealthy ideas and separate them from the healthy ones. It is about turning those unhealthy beliefs into healthy ones.

Healthy ideas are rational and unhealthy ones are irrational. You will learn, if you do the exercises in this chapter, how to differentiate your thoughts and how to change your thinking. Most people who do the work suggested in this chapter have these immediate results:

1. Their personalities improve.

2. Their natural happiness increases.

3. Their ability to cope with difficulties increases.

4. Their new beliefs about conception and carrying a healthy baby to full term enable them to feel safer and more hopeful.

The Rational Thought Process (RTP)

Irrational thinking can have an enormously negative impact on fertility. If you are hoping to conceive, you can aid that process by exploring how your thoughts may be blocking your path to complete mind/body potential and fertility. In this chapter, you will learn how to let rational thoughts emerge and dominate your behavior. Once you learn how to think rationally, the tendency to let irrational thinking cause havoc in your life at first lessens and then disappears.

Through our thoughts, we make ourselves feel the way we feel. With the information and beliefs which we currently have at any given moment, however, we may not be able to change how we feel. For example, if you feel powerless and hopeless about conception at this time, you may be unable to make yourself feel any other way. After learning and applying the new information in this chapter, however, you will be able to make yourself feel different. As a patient of the well-known practitioner of mind/body medicine, Dr. Bernie Siegel, said, "I make my own weather—today it's sunny all day."

To achieve positive thinking and rationality, I use several techniques. First and foremost is the Rational Thought Process (RTP), which is based on the method developed by the internationally known Professor of Psychiatry, Maxie Maultsby, M.D. I had the good fortune of working with Dr. Maultsby and learning his method when we were both working at the Simonton Cancer Center in California. He taught his method to patients who were afraid of dying, helping them turn fear into serenity. I've discovered that his method works equally well with women and men who are dealing with the fear of not being able to conceive and carry a healthy baby to full term.

Before we learn how to use the Rational Thought Process, however, we have to understand irrational thinking and thought disorders. We need to know the nature of our illness before we can understand and apply the cure.

How To Begin

Remember that the goal of this chapter is to identify and change any thought processes which may be inhibiting fertility. Your thinking may be causing negative emotions, and the way to change those negative emotions is to change your thinking. Start by taking the following actions:

1. Take out a sheet of paper and list all of your ideas and behaviors, which seem natural and normal to you, but which are self-defeating and likely related to pregnancy, conception, motherhood or fatherhood.

For example:

A. Smoking cigarettes, which I do many times a day, is unhealthy and self-defeating.

B. Working fourteen hours a day is my normal schedule and its not healthy.

C. My normal fast food eating behaviors are not healthy.

D. The thoughts I often have that I'll never get pregnant, that I've tried too many times, that I don't deserve to have a baby, that I'm being punished for the abortion I had when I was very young are unhealthy thoughts.

2. Use the examples in the next section on Rational Thought to learn how to write out corresponding healthier, rational beliefs. At first, these healthy beliefs may seem unnatural and abnormal to you.

3. Keep a copy of your list of healthy beliefs with you at all times.

4. Read all of the new healthy beliefs daily until they seem normal and natural to you.

5. Read the corresponding healthy beliefs every time one of the old unhealthy beliefs surfaces in your mind.

6. Continue to practice these new beliefs and behaviors until they become natural and normal for you.

Characteristics of Rational Thought

It is easier to move in the direction of fertility, pregnancy, and parenthood if you move your thoughts in the direction of the "rational." Rational thoughts are thoughts based on reality and not on emotions, particularly not on fear-based emotions. Here are some examples of the characteristics of rational thoughts and corresponding irrational thoughts:

1. Rational thoughts are true, and based on objective reality.

Thinking that is not true
We don't deserve to get pregnant. Perhaps it is right that we have not gotten pregnant because a baby could ruin our career, our marriage and our lives.

Thinking that is true
We have tried to get pregnant with or without professional help and we are still not pregnant. Only we can ruin our careers, our marriage and our lives.

2. Rational thoughts help protect your life and your health.

Thinking that is not healthy
A baby will drain me of all my energy. I'll be sucked dry.

Thinking that is healthy
There are many things that I can
do to preserve my energy if I
choose. A baby can bring great
joy and that can be energizing.

3. Rational thoughts help you to attain your goals.

*Thinking that does not lead to
your goals*
I want a baby but I don't want to change my eating, alcohol, nicotine or
pot habits. I don't want to change my so-called stressful way of life.

Thinking that does lead to your goals

I don't feel like changing my habits of eating and using alcohol and pot,
or my stressful way of life, but I really want to conceive and want to
carry a healthy baby to term, so I'll change one step at a time.

4. Rational thoughts are positive and keep you from feeling the way you don't want to feel.

Thinking that makes you feel bad
I have no experience with babies.I'll be an awful parent.

Thinking that helps you to feel better
It's true that I have no experience, but I can take a class and discuss ideas on child rearing with my spouse. I can read on the subject. I can develop my own ideas of what I think a good parent is and try to become that.

5. Rational thoughts keep you out of unwanted trouble with your spouse, friends and family.

Thinking that gets you into trouble
I don't think my husband will participate in our child's life or be a good parent.

Thinking that doesn't get you
                    into trouble
I can ask my husband what plans he has for participating in our child's life. His answer may surprise me. We can discuss together how we plan to parent our child.

How to Achieve Rational Thought Through the Rational Thought Process

Now that you have made a list of your unhealthy and healthy beliefs and you understand the nature of rational thoughts, you can use a step-by-step format for changing irrational and negative thoughts that arise in specific situations into positive, rational ones. Try this. It works.

1.   Write down all the facts about a situation or event which make you feel anxious.

Example: Antoinette's Story—My father sent me to boarding school when I was ten years old. He didn't spend much time with me.

When he was with me he was only physically present, not emotionally. He wasn't a father to me.

2.   Now read your account and delete or change anything that is not a fact.

Example: He wasn't a father to me.

Change it to the truth: He is my biological father.

3.   Write down all the thoughts you have about the facts you have just written.

Example: I thought that the reason my father sent me away was because I did something wrong. I thought that the reason he didn't spend much time with me was because I wasn't likable or lovable. I thought I was preventing my father from doing what he needed to do. I thought that the reason he was not emotionally present was because I wasn't important.

4.   Write down your feelings about the facts in #1.

Example: I felt angry, scared, confused and abandoned when my father sent me to boarding school. I felt ashamed around my friends because my father didn't spend time with me. When he was only present physically and not emotionally, I felt very lonely and depressed.

5.   Now change the thoughts in #3 to positive, truthful rational thoughts.

Example:

There are people who like me and love me. There are people who enjoy spending time with me. I enjoy spending time with me.

My father sent me away to school for his own reasons which possibly had nothing to do with me. I have heard from others that my father was rarely emotionally present. My father's not being emotionally present with me has nothing to do with whether I am important or not.

I choose not to be like my father. I make a conscious choice to be emotionally present with my children, spouse and friends.

If someone treats me the same way my father did, I can choose not to feel responsible for his/her behavior.

6.   Write an affirmation which incorporates these rational thoughts.

Example: Just because my father didn't know how to father me emotionally doesn't mean that I can't learn how to father/mother my own child emotionally.

7.   Write a plan of action.

Example: I will learn how to be a good father/mother by talking with people whom I think are good parents or who felt they had good fathers. I will take a parenting class and will read literature on the subject. I will observe my child's reactions to my parenting. I will listen to my child, talk with my child and ask what he/she wants and needs from me.

As you can see from the above steps, the Rational Thought Process is based on becoming aware of:

A.   What we perceive through our senses (what we see, hear, taste, smell and feel physically).

B.   Our thoughts about those perceptions.

C.   Our emotional reactions to those thoughts.

Using the following example of Ann and Arthur, we can see how this works.

Ann and Arthur

Ann and Arthur, did an RTP which revealed and then changed their thinking patterns. Here is what they discovered in the process:

A. Ann sees a baby nursing.

B. She thinks, "Oh that baby is so sweet and that mother looks so content. I really want to have a baby and be a mother."

C. These positive thoughts make Ann feel good about the baby and about motherhood.

Explanation. Ann's thoughts and beliefs about event (A)—seeing a mother nursing her baby—lead to her feelings at (C), her decision to become a mother.

Here, however, is Arthur's reaction to the same event:

A. Arthur sees a woman nursing a baby.

B. Arthur thinks they look so involved with each other that there appears to be no room for anyone else. "I would feel left out if it were my spouse and baby," Arthur believes.

C. Arthur's thoughts of feeling left out make him decide that he doesn't want to share his wife with a baby.

Explanation. Arthur's thoughts about having a baby and his not being able to discuss these feelings may have led to his having decreased sperm motility.

Now here are Arthur's thoughts after doing an RTP and discussing it:

A.   Arthur sees a woman nursing a baby.

B.   Arthur thinks they look very involved with each other. Now he thinks, "I would like to be that involved with a baby. I could be that involved. I could give my spouse a break and feed our baby one bottle of pumped breast milk daily. I'd like to be a father."

C.   Arthur's new thoughts about having a baby make him happy and secure and can even increase the motility of his sperm.

By changing his irrational, fearful thoughts in (B), he changes his entire outlook on having a child and being a father. His new positive thoughts helped produce physical changes necessary for conception.

Here are two more examples of women and men who have successfully used the Rational Thought Process:

Anna

Anna, 27 years-old, in great health, wanted very much to have a baby. She was referred to me because there seemed to be no reasonable explanation for why she was not conceiving. She was a very warm and outgoing young woman who appeared not to have a care in the world. I first met with Anna and her husband, and their relationship seemed supportive and loving. I then saw Anna alone over a period of three months. I discovered that she had learned how to mask her feelings well, not when she was a child, as she came from a loving expressive family, but sometime in her young adulthood. The only problem she talked about, however, was an uneasiness with her mother-in-law. One day I asked her to imagine pregnancy from conception to birth. During the labor imagery she began to cry. She said there was something which she had not told anyone. One night, about eight years ago, six years before she married, Anna had been raped while walking across her college campus. She hadn't told a soul, not even her husband. We spoke of this for several weeks and Anna agreed to go to a rape crisis center. She then agreed to write out an RTP.

Slowly she began to feel better, safer and no longer guilty. She was able to tell her husband and her sister about the rape. She found she could play more and work more efficiently and less compulsively. Her relationship with her husband became carefree. She started to feel at ease with her mother-in-law. Within one year Anna was able to conceive naturally and to have a healthy vaginal birth.

Pete

Pete, a 32 year-old lawyer, came to the clinic because he and his spouse, Rori, 31, also a lawyer, had been trying to get pregnant for the past year and a half. With a diagnosis of low sperm count and motility, which is usually due both to stress and dietary practices which are rich in extremes, Pete was the designated patient. Rori was not hopeful about Pete's ability to work a holistically oriented program. Although she had insisted that he come to the clinic, she still felt that it wouldn't work—his sperm would never be able to penetrate her egg.

Pete, meanwhile, felt disempowered by Rori's attitude toward him and resentful toward her. He had been working longer and longer hours and more and more days so that they barely saw each other. After dealing with many childhood issues surrounding his father, Pete began to understand his relationship with Rori better. He asked for a couples session, during which time he discussed creating a proper environment for conception to occur. They each agreed to spend at least one evening a week together from six o'clock on with the phone turned off. They also agreed to go away one weekend a month. They each drew a picture of the sperm and the ovum meeting. In Rori's drawing, the penetration of the egg was simple.

Both Rori and Pete asked themselves, "What do I need to do to move in the direction of pregnancy?" and both found the same answer—to spend more meaningful time together. They each agreed that they needed to become emotionally supportive of each other. Rori promised not to sabotage the progress which Pete was making. They both did an RTP around their negative beliefs and they not only kept a copy of their own RTP, but each had a copy of the other's. They began to eat a healthier diet, to walk together four times a week for twenty minutes and to continue to explore the ambivalence in their marriage -not about having a child—but about the feeling they each had that they were not getting enough nurturing from the other. How could they possibly nurture a child until they learned how to nurture themselves and each other?

After four months, Pete's sperm count and motility were normal. He was thrilled. After eight months in the program, Rori and Pete conceived and Rori carried their healthy baby girl to full term.

It is very important to your success for you to write out an RTP for each problem or issue. When you have completed your RTP, read it aloud to at least one other person. Then be sure to read it to yourself at least twice a week for the next three weeks. By doing this you are retraining the way your brain thinks on certain issues.

For many people, this empowering but time consuming exercise is hard to accept, much less to do. Our culture has trained us to want the quick-fix, the instant cure, the aspirin-for-headache, Prozac-for-depression approach to illness. Thus many people prefer to go directly to In Vitro Fertilization (IVF), Gamete Intra-FallopianTransfer (Gift), or Zygote IntraFallopian Transfer(Zift). It seems easier to spend thousands of dollars on new technology than to spend time building a new way of thinking. This is unfortunate, however, because many couples still need to do an RTP and the other exercises in this book in order to allow the techniques of reproductive medicine to be effective and successful. A healthy outlook needs to be present for the technology to work—its called integrative medicine. There is no magic. As in all other things, success requires hard work.

Now it's your turn. Good luck with writing your own Rational Thought Process and congratulations on taking the first step towards being present for yourself in a new and healthier way.

Chapter Four

Creative Healing

The fertility of your reproductive system can be increased as you develop certain parts of your personality. What hidden qualities need to be allowed to emerge or at least acknowledged before you can bring forth life? In order to conceive, we all need to connect to the feminine parts of our personality, the center of all life. We also need to respect the parts of our psyche that lead us to our passion.

It is also important to utilize all of what we have in healing. We used the rational in Chapter 2. Now we will use the non-rational, the intuitive side, in meditation and imagery. In this modern age, we are steeped in technology. The "woman's way of knowing and healing" has not been socially and politically respected as it was in the past, but we, as women, need to begin to respect our own nature. The exercises in this chapter will help us do so.

To become aware of the unknown and seemingly non-existent parts of your personality, each member of a couple hoping to conceive should start by honestly asking him or herself some questions:

1. What needs of mine are not being met?

2. How can I meet these needs more consistently?

3. Do I need to develop the parts of my personality which can meet these needs before we conceive?

4. Is it realistic to expect a baby to give our lives the meaning that we have not yet been able to give to ourselves?

The goal of this entire program is to touch the healer within and the techniques in this chapter are an important step in reaching that goal.

A Note on Time:

To become aware of the purpose of your own life takes persistence, and time—meaning sustained attention. This is often difficult, particularly when you have already been trying to get pregnant for a long time. I don't have any more time, you say. I have the desire and the will but not the time. Mechanistic methods seem easier. It appears faster to remain separate from your body, from your own relationship to your fertility and to let technology impregnate you. True healing, however, and real fertility, requires that you experience the intensity of your unconscious fears, needs, desires and infinite capacities. You must develop a new relation to the "1" of you, to the essence of your personality, the self beneath your persona, beneath the pretenses. If you take the time to get in touch with your own natural rhythm, you will soon become responsive to your own normal needs and desires.

Time is necessary to give your body the attention it needs. Sickness forces you to do so, but there are certainly better ways of giving the body attention. Decide now, if you choose, to give your body/mind the attention it deserves to restore, health and balance. You have one life to lead. What do you want to do with it? Write spontaneously whatever comes to your mind for 5 minutes. Write your wildest desires and dreams. See who you really are.

What Do I Really Want to Do with My Time?

Meditation

Meditation is "letting go." It is creating a stillness of the mind and a release of all thoughts as we enter the light beyond the mind. It is a state in which the heart is open and the mind is clear. In this state, we allow our own true nature to emerge. Through meditation, our old ways of experiencing the world melt away, permitting new knowledge, new awareness, new questions and a new opening of body pathways.

We use meditation for infertility to reduce stress and tension and to quiet the mind. When the mind is quiet, it is more awake and aware. In this state of mental and physical relaxation, there are changes in brain wave patterns and an increase in cerebral blood flow. Regular meditation enables the body to metabolize serotonin, which in turn can affect the metabolism of oxygen radicals, those unstable molecules which can damage the energy and intelligence of our cells. This damage to our cells helps cause aging, heart disease, cancer, arthritis and infertility. Meditation enhances the body's natural defenses against disease. An example of this was shown in a study published in the journal SCI-ENCE, August, 1996. The study found that Transcendental Meditation (TM) was twice as effective in lowering the blood pressure of African-American men and women as progressive muscle relaxation and instruction on healthier living habits, two other frequently recommended non-medical methods of reducing stress. Not only did TM do a better job, 80% of the study participants were still practicing it five years after the study concluded.

Stress is not a result of the process of trying to conceive—it is our reaction to that process. In most cases of unexplained infertility, it can take as long as seven months to conceive. During that time, individuals experiencing this "crisis" are mobilized for a "fight or flight" response. There is no let up of this natural response of our body until a couple has conceived and the energy triggered by the adrenal and pituitary hormones is dissipated or discharged. This constant stress can weaken the immune system, and every pregnancy interacts with the maternal immune system.

The brain is our main organ of comfort and survival, and meditation works to calm the mind and automatically directs the therapeutic change to other organs. In meditation, we let go of all past learning, all old beliefs and attitudes and all present thoughts. Consistently practiced, it can help you attain a mental, physical and spiritual comfort zone.

Thoughts on meditation for Fertility

In meditation "you see with the heart; what is essential is invisible to the mind" (The Little Prince, Antoine de Saint-Exupéry) There is a realization that comes about in meditation that there is a oneness that we in this world share. Being silent with yourself and being silent with your invitation to your baby deepens both your positive experience of fertility treatments. Meditation opens our frantic lives and demanding schedules to a pleasant harmony. Meditation can provide you with a necessary silent respite on a daily basis along with an interim renewal and an opening of your heart to love.

I live in California and meet many people who talk about meditation and read books on meditation and go to lectures on meditation* The only way to learn how to meditate is the same way you learn how to play tennis or ride a bike or learn to read. Practice, practice, practice. In meditation it is sit, sit, sit—focus, focus, focus. The technique of meditation is very simple—sit in a comfortable position with your spine straight and your feet flat on the floor. Close your eyes. Breathe normally. Recite a mantra, your mind cleansing word silently to yourself. A common mantra is: MA RA NA THA—an Aramaic phrase that means Come Lord. If that feels too religious to you, choose a more secular

---

* They are interested in meditation and are willing to gather information about meditation and they often find it difficult to begin and to maintain the practice.

mantra such as: PA CEM MA. Once you have your mantra it is a good idea to keep it rather than changing it

After sitting in your position comfortably, close your eyes and recite your mantra silently over and over and over and over again for 5 minutes. The optimum time and a reasonably attainable goal is 2 sittings daily for 20 minutes. However, in order to succeed, begin with one sitting daily for 5 minutes and gradually increase the number of minutes and sittings. The purpose of starting slowing is to assure your success i.e. make the goal easier to meet than not to meet.

What you will probably experience since we humans are all very similar is a barrage of thoughts and mental chatter, a monkey mind of sorts: this is none of your business, your only task is to sit as still as possible and to continually repeat your mantra over and over and over. The thoughts will come and go, old feelings may emerge, they too will come and go—continue repeating your mantra -past hurts and happiness', longings, hopes, dreams, mundane tasks, shopping lists, annoyances, garbage trucks outside, car alarms, telephones all will attempt to intrude on this time. None of this is important none of this needs your attention—continue like a broken record to repeat your mantra to yourself over and over and over. This is all you do when you meditate. Ancient memories that you thought you had forgotten, maybe even horrible memories of child abuse, assault, rape, other kinds of brutality may emerge. Do not try to stop those thoughts or tears or memories. Allow them to come. Do not try to hold onto them, allow them to go. They have a life of their own, they will follow their own path and pattern. Your work is to continue repeating your mantra during this mental storm.

As a counterpart, you may see a blue light or a white light or multi-colored lights, you may see or recall things that make your laugh, you may experience a feeling of deep peace and bliss. Once again pay no mind to these feelings and thoughts. They too need to come and go as they please, not as you please. For you, please just continue repeating your mantra.

Meditation will give you a deep sense of freedom and yet a sense of community. Imagine if all the fertility mothers of the world began to meditate two times a day. What an amazing way to create harmony and understanding for yourself and the world. What an amazing way to renew the life of your spiritual self and to connect to your desired baby. Meditation erases the veil of confusion and illusion. We can see clearly and in the process release our cares and concerns. Meditation illuminates our way of seeing. In meditation we can enter into the stream of infinity, the boundless and the absolute.

Meditation is washing your mind out with a verbal toothbrush. So now, if you will:

Choose a chair and a room and a time for your daily meditation. Write it on your calendar. Make a date with yourself. This will probably be the greatest exploration and tradition you will ever establish in your life.

Now write your ambivalence below about beginning your meditation practice and then begin it anyway. Resistance is normal. We are all creatures of habit. We as women can change the world—can create peace.

In an experiment in a crime-ridden neighborhood in Washington, D.C.(not the hill). A group of meditators did their work of meditation 2 times a day for peace. After 1 month the crime rate was statistically significantly lowered.*

If you don't like the idea of a mantra, you may of course just sit and focus on your breath. Do not consciously alter your breathing in any way just observe it and observe it and observe it. The thoughts will come as they do with any meditation, follow the same path as with the mantra letting the thoughts come and go.

Keep increasing your time gradually. The form never changes. It is a consistent, lovely ritual to do in the middle of the chaos of modern life. After doing this practice, you will begin to see and feel many benefits. It

---

* See T.M. Study www.mapi.com

will bring you such deep rewards that you will probably choose to make it a part of your life for all time. It is free, pleasurable, life enhancing, joy producing and energizing. All it takes is practice and a commitment to do it. There is nothing esoteric about meditation. You do not have to be religious and, if you are, it will not interfere with your religious beliefs and practices. You do not have to be spiritual, an airhead, a vegetarian or a guru. There are no restrictions and no requirements other than that you do it. The rest will take care of itself. It usually takes at least three months to make meditation a habitual part of your life, so please don't give up. It may be the most important thing you will ever do for yourself. You deserve the peace, creativity and joy that silencing your mind every day can bring.

Meditation is not the same as listening to music, reading a book, playing an instrument, watching TV or hanging out on the computer. It cannot be compared to anything else. It takes commitment, discipline, being gentle with yourself and being detached from the outcome. I used to work in an alcohol and drug treatment center and remember the words of coke addict after coke addict about meditation: "It is the only thing that surpasses cocaine at its best. It is not like coke in any way but it makes me so clear and so naturally high that I never want to quit doing it." If meditation can center someone whose mind was toyed with by cocaine, it can probably center anyone.

Meditation can promote healing, increase relaxation and remove some of the deep-seated causes that block physical energy.

What is Imagery:

Imagery is a form of intentional relaxation and mental direction. It is a technique for forming mental images around desired outcomes in life. Imagination affects our lives and our bodies in many amazing ways. Recall the scent of your first perfume or your lovers and you may be flooded with a biochemistry of emotions and other connected memories. Recall the scent of a lilac or an orange blossom and other emotions will be linked.

Imagine yourself being told you must speak in front of a large group of people on a subject not in your field. Many changes in your body will probably occur. You may become flushed and sweaty with a rise in blood pressure, your brain waves will change and you may feel a bit feint. Now imagine yourself being told you must speak on a subject that you enjoy. You have one month to prepare. All the research has been done for you. You will be paid substantially to prepare and to present. Go a bit further and see yourself having completed this month of preparation and you are halfway through the lecture, the audience is intrigued and you feel confident and playful. You come to the end and there is great applause and much interest. All of these happenings are just the workings of your imagination, yet each one has the ability to affect your biochemistry and your emotions in different ways. We learn and remember through our senses—sight, taste, touch, hearing, smell and movement. For our purpose, imagery is a way of thinking that uses the senses to communicate the desired emotion to affect a bodily change and a more hopeful outcome.

Imagery helps us alter old images of expected outcomes. We cannot lie to our body. Our body immediately registers what we experience through our senses or what it experiences through our mind (if I can for a moment make that bifurcation of the body/mind). In the exercises in this chapter, we will use imagined rehearsals of fertility procedures, processes and outcomes as an integral part of establishing electrochem-ical pathways that translate thoughts into physiological changes.

We will also use tools to enhance imagery, including hypnosis, music, aromatherapy, drawing, writing out the visualization and reading it aloud. All of these tools and techniques will be explained and sample imagery scripts will be given to you.

Imagery and Visualization

Visualization was first introduced in the treatment of illness by 0. Carl Simonton, M.D., a radiation oncologist. Along with conventional cancer therapies, Dr. Simonton taught his patients how to use visualization for self-healing. After working with Dr. Simonton for ten years and seeing how effective visualization, along with hypnosis and meditation were for seriously ill patients in their healing, I decided to use it with fertility patients.

Imagery utilizes all the senses. Since we learn through our senses, we can communicate through imagery with our bodies in order to bring about emotional and physiological modifications. Alterations in thought and emotions can actually change the autonomic functions of the body—those involuntary activities such as breathing, heart rate, and blood pressure. Both negative states of mind and positive mental images can affect the immune system. If we can participate in our illness, we can certainly participate in our healing.

The Biology of Imagery

As said before, every pregnancy interacts with the maternal immune system. The pituitary gland and the hypothalamus are connected to each other chemically and neurally, which explains how the hypothalamus alters the hormonal systems of the body. Hormones not only act on the ovaries and testes but also on every cell in the body.

The important point here is that every thought and emotion has a neuroanatomical bridge to the body. The mind/body responds as a unit, since every thought has a biochemical and electrochemical action. What's more, the image we have of something can have as much of an effect as the thing itself. For example, if during labor a woman feels stressed because of some negative thought that has entered her mind, her brain waves are altered, her endorphins—the body's natural painkillers—are depleted, and the production of catecholamines are stimulated, further blocking the remaining endorphins. As a result, she feels increased pain.

In order to move in the direction of fertile thinking, we need to address not only the biological but also the social and psychological aspects of your diagnosis and how all these elements interact with each other. Imagery not only helps change your physiology, it also aids in giving you a feeling of control over your adaptive responses, allowing you to decrease your fear and anxiety. Most significantly, it helps you understand that fertile thinking is important to all aspects of your life. This kind of creative thinking permits the potential for positive change in all your body systems—most particularly, your reproductive system.

The new fertility technology often puts the focus on the procedures themselves, or on the diagnosis for the insurance company, rather than on the couple. Remember that the purpose of all your treatments is to bring a new life into this world. It is about joy. And it is about you as a couple. Whatever the problem, it is usually difficult to attribute it solely to one or the other of you. It is best to regard it, both physiologically and emotionally, as a couple situation. All of the exercises in this book are for both partners, no matter what the diagnosis. Albert Schweitzer said, "We all have within us a wise physician.!' Unhealthy thinking can interfere with ovulation, cause tubal spasms, upset menstrual cycles, and effect sperm motility. Medicine cannot improve on Mother Nature at her best. Decide to participate in your own fertility with your mind, your body and your spirit. The essence of healing is directing your energy to your own advantage. You can then set in motion the divine healer within.

How to Use Visualization and Imagery

Begin by looking at the word INFERTILITY. Then, spontaneously, write answers to these questions:

1. What are your thoughts, expectations and images surrounding infertility?

2. Within the context of your own belief system, what is your understanding of your diagnosis? What images do you have surrounding the statistics of your condition? Write down whatever comes to mind.

INFERILITY

Now look at the word FERTILITY. Free associate—write down your beliefs and thoughts—the first things that come into your mind—about fertility.

Free associate to the word: CONCEPTION

Free associate to the word: PREGNANCY

From these negative and positive images you have written, you can now create a specific imagery that is right for you.

EXAMPLE: INFERTILITY is dark, hopeless, black, empty.

FERTILITY is light, joyous, green, blossoming.

Step 1: Using crayons or colored pencils, draw a picture of INFERTILITY and then tear it up, crumple it, burn it, or discard it in any way you choose.

Step 2: Draw a picture of FERTILTY; Draw a hopeful picture, e.g. something light, joyous, green and blossoming.

Step 3: Sit in your meditation position and close your eyes. Breathe in through your nose and exhale as slowly as you can through your mouth, sending your breath all the way down your spine. Contract all the muscles in your body from your feet to your forehead and then release them. Feel the tension flow out of your body and into the ground. Then begin a guided imagery of your own along the lines of the following:

Feel your right arm growing very heavy, your jaw relaxed, your eyelids very, very heavy. Imagine a gentle spring breeze filled with the scent of freshly mowed grass flowing across your abdomen and into your uterus and Fallopian tubes. Imagine your ovaries filled with a healing white light. Feel a deep sense of joy flowing through your belly. As you begin to feel very peaceful, imagine you have a piece of chalk in one hand and an eraser in the other. In front of you is a blank slate. Write the number 10, draw a circle around it, and erase it. Slowly do the same thing with a 9, then 8, 7, 6, 5, 4, 3, 2, 1. When you have erased all the numbers, you will be in a state of deep inner peace and in touch with the wondrous fertility of nature and the grand fertility of your own way of being.

Now, imagine yourself standing on the sandy bank of a safe and beautiful lake. It is so shallow you could wade across it if you chose. From where you stand you can see every part of the lake. On the shore is a boat waiting just for you. It has everything you need to be comfortable.

You move the boat by willing it to go wherever you want. When it comes to you, you step into it and find a comfortable place to sit and relax. Close your eyes and just drift. Listen to the sounds of nature—to the birds, the crickets, the frogs. Imagine a healing white light entering through the top of your skull. It flows throughout your body, into your chest and extremities. You feel a love and compassion for yourself deeper than you have felt in a long, long time. You float and you see darkness, hopelessness, fear and any idea that you have of infertility. Let them grow as large as possible and then shrink them to the size of a pinpoint. You see these images leaving your body and going off into the sky in balloons of release. Watch them until they disappear. Now direct your boat to a beautiful cove surrounded by a grassy bank and lovely wildflowers. Here you await your own inner fertility guide. It may take any form—a person, an animal, a feather, or just a voice. When you feel its presence, ask whatever question you want. A common question is: What do I need to do to get pregnant? Relax and wait for the answer. Before you leave your trance, ask your guide to meet with you whenever you choose. Conjure up a healing fertility image for yourself and decide to use that image every day. Now start counting up from 1 and at the count of 5 you will be wide awake, refreshed, relaxed and filled with renewed hope. Your eyes are no longer heavy. Your right arm is no longer heavy. Take a deep awakening breath. Your eyes are wide open. Your head is totally clear and you can perform all of your activities safely and serenely.

You can now visualize the imagery you decided on in your trance in an awake state. This usually takes only a minute. It is a good idea to do this at least once a day and to do the entire guided imagery once a week. Have fun with this, take your time, be patient with yourself, and do not ignore the answers you receive. This is not something to be taken lightly. Respect the healer within you.

Some people find it difficult to do a guided imagery because they are overwhelmed with the stress of everyday life and of trying to become pregnant. I suggest that you write out your imagery and make a few copies. Keep one in your wallet. Take it out frequently and read it aloud or silently to yourself. I also suggest that, along with your drawing of infertility, you write out a statement about infertility, such as:

> "I have many thoughts, emotions, and images about infertility. I must acknowledge their existence and give them verbal expression so they do not seek expression through my body. I take charge of these feelings and dissipate them. There are many areas in my life in which I am very fertile. I am having some difficulty conceiving, or my spouse is, and I will participate in getting my body and my mind prepared for conception and pregnancy in every healthy way I know. (Your husband's name or sperm donor's name) sperm and my egg actually want to meet each other. When they do meet and his sperm fertilizes my egg, our resulting embryo will easily implant in my uterus and become a developing fetus. I'll have a successful pregnancy, an easy vaginal birth and a beautiful, healthy baby."

Whenever you begin to have repeated negative thoughts immediately take out this paper and read it aloud to yourself. Each partner in the relationship ought to have a copy so that if one of you is unable to help yourself, the other can read it aloud in a loving and caring way. Again, be gentle with yourself. You want to reduce your stress level, not increase it. Invite the soul of your baby into your calm, healthy body.

Imagery and Fertility:

Your own negative-spontaneous imagery reflects the unconscious attitudes you hold around your fertility. To further explore this, draw another picture, in color, of the sperm attempting to reach the ovum and draw or write in the obstacles that he (sperm) encounters. Please do this without editing your thoughts and feelings and have your spouse or partner do the same.

Example of Man's drawing: Obstacles between the egg and the sperm.

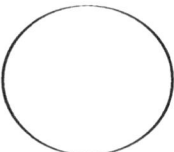

I don't have enough money to take care of you and our baby the way I think I should.

Sex will be the last thing on your mind.
You'll have no more time for me.
You'll be nursing the baby and we'll never be alone
Once you become a mother you'll forget about playing and traveling

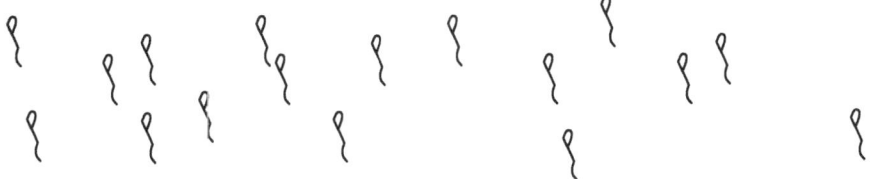

Example of a Woman's drawing: Obstacles between the egg and the sperm.

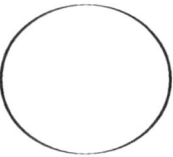

This is hopeless

My cells are disorganized

My egg and your sperm are working against each other. They are angry with each other.

What will happen to my career?

You'll have an affair if I get fat.

I am not a person I am just a cycle.

You want the children raised in your religion and I don't know how I'll tell my family.

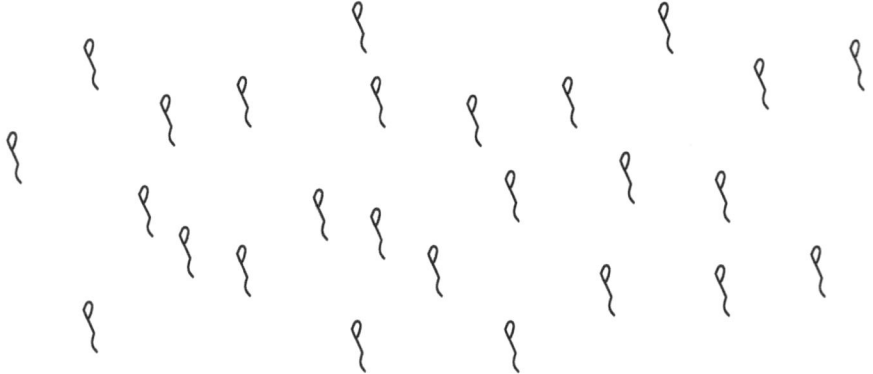

Male—Obstacles between eggs and sperm

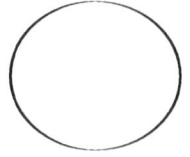

Female—Obstacles between eggs and sperm

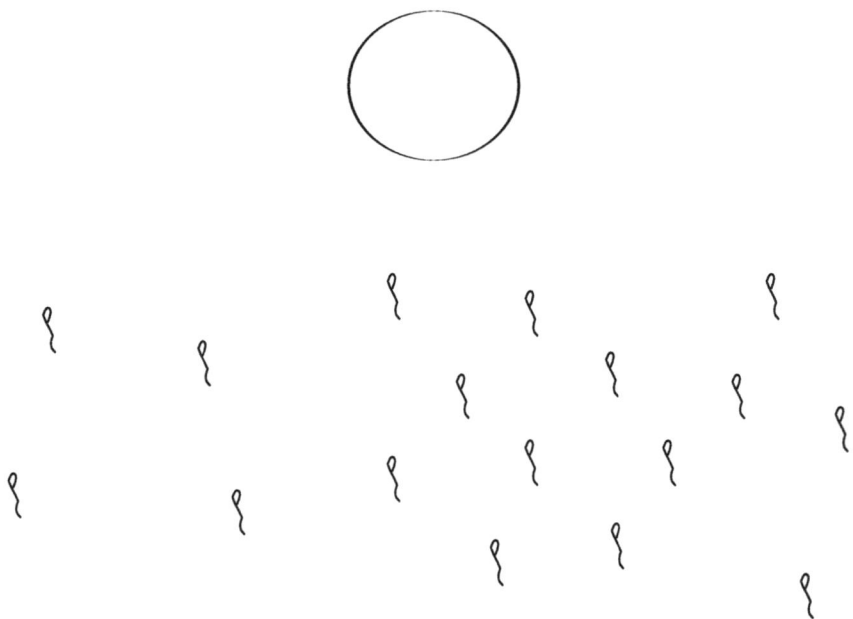

Woman: Now draw a picture, in color, of the sperm and egg meeting without any obstacles. It can be a symbolic drawing. Be creative. Play with it. Have Fun.

Man: Now draw a picture, in color, of sperm and egg meetingwithout any obstacles. It can be a symbolic drawing. Be creative. Play with it. Have Fun.

Hypnosis

A good way to stay in the present during the practice of your imagery is to use self-hypnosis. Hypnosis is an altered state of consciousness and physiologic calm. It is a normal state that occurs just as you are drifting into sleep. Since hypnosis is a naturally occurring physiological state that all people experience right before falling asleep, everyone can be hypnotized. Not everyone will allow themselves to be hypnotized and some are resistant to it. If you are resistant to hypnosis, the first step is to understand why you are resistant by exploring your beliefs and fears and the myths surrounding hypnosis. The second step is to practice, practice, practice.

All hypnosis is really self hypnosis. The hypnotist is merely a facilitator in the process. You have to be willing to accept the hypnotic script and to participate in the process. Without your willing participation hypnosis cannot occur. Hypnosis works through suggestions. Our minds are constantly given suggestive stimuli, both from the external world and from our internal world. These suggestions have created both our good and bad habits, our ability to relax ourselves and stress ourselves. In hypnosis we attempt to replace the negative stimuli with positive stimuli. If we see the mind, the body, the spirit and our emotions as a quartet, then maybe we can see that a harmonious arrangement is beneficial. When the mind and spirit are peaceful, the body feels good and we experience pleasurable emotions. These pleasurable emotions and reduction in anxiety help to maintain the body's equilibrium

Using one or more of the following scripts, we can now begin a regular program of self-hypnosis and guided imagery.
Schedule:

> Day I: Read one of the following scripts aloud to yourself. Follow all the suggestions (except, of course, the suggestion to close your eyes). Purchase a cassette tape.

Day II: Record the script in the third person on your cassette tape. Read it aloud as slowly as possible pausing frequently for 15 seconds.

Day III: Select a regular place and time for listening to your tape. Find a comfortable place and position. Turn the phone off and the answering machine all the way down.

You may order the tapes in the back of the book, if you choose not to make your own.

Script 1: Natural Conception

Get yourself into a comfortable position and begin to observe what is in front of you. Now take a deep breath through your nose, filling your abdomen with air. Feel it blowing up like a balloon. Good. Now as slowly as you possibly can exhale through your mouth and send the breath all the way down your spine…. Now, just focus on your next three exhalations. Don't alter them in any way. Just observe them. Well done…. Now contract your feet and your ankles…. and gently release them. Contract your calves, your shins and your knees…. and relax them. Take another deep breath in through your nose…. and exhale as slowly as you can through your mouth, sending the breath into your right great toe…. Contract your thighs…. and relax them. Inhale through your nose…exhale as slowly as you can through your mouth, sending the breath into your left great toe…. Focus on your exhalations…. Now turn your attention to your abdomen and all of its contents, including your reproductive system. Become aware of all the feelings that you hold in this area….Label these feelings as a point of reference, but not in judgment. Now take a deep healing breath and breathe all of the feelings out of your abdomen. You can always deal with them at another time. They have no place in a body that is trying to relax. Inhale deeply and breathe out, sending all of your feelings way out into the universe…. Again take a deep healing breath and release your feelings sending them way out into the universe…Now contract your chest and your shoulders and relax them…Contract your right arm and your left arm. Make a fist with your hands and now extend them and let them relax and fall wherever they are comfortable. Now contract your spine until your entire back is arched with tension, and release it. Good…. and take a deep healing breath and send it all the way down your spine…. Contract your face, your jaw, scrunch it up like a prune…. and now open your mouth and your eyes as wide as you can, stick out your tongue and try to touch your chin. Imagine that you are an animal in the wild and that you are releasing your energy through a grand stretch of your body and a great release of sound from deep within your being. Now feel your entire body letting go to the force of gravity. Now imagine yourself climbing down a stairwell that leads to a lovely small lake. Count yourself down 10 relaxing, 9…, 8…, feeling very peaceful…, 7…, 6…deeper now, 5…. Letting go of all unnecessary tension, 4, deeper and deeper, 3, and down, 2, and deeper and deeper and down, one…and down. Now you are at the shore of your own personal lake of healing. It is a lovely spring day. The temperature is perfect. It is midday and the sun is almost directly overhead. There is a gentle breeze and you can hear the soft sounds of nature and you can smell the sweet scents of all the flowers and the lush green foliage. From every point on this lake you can see it in its entirety. You could even walk across it if you chose. The water comes up only to your waist. At the shore, a boat is ready and waiting for you. It is complete, with everything on it that you might need for your satisfaction and comfort. You can move the boat by willing it to go wherever you choose. You climb onto it and settle yourself into a relaxed position. You float and you dream, and float and dream. Now you will yourself over to the cove of healing. From here you can see all a myriad of wildflowers and the grand old trees shading the cove. There is a creek trickling down into the lake and its sound soothes you even more. You are very relaxed and feel very safe and peaceful. You decide to ask your own inner wisdom, "what do I need to do to get pregnant?"…And you wait for an answer.

If you don't get an answer this time, you will eventually, perhaps the next time you do this relaxation. If you do get an answer decide to follow through and respect the information. Now you are in a receptive state and ready to begin your imagery.

IMAGERY I

It is easy for me to get pregnant. I see myself conceiving at my next ovulation.

My ovum easily releases from the lutenizing follicle and passes through my ovarian wall. Now, the fimbria at the end of my fallopian tube sweep my egg into my tube. Meanwhile, my fertile cervical fluid is directing the healthy sperm through my cervix into my fallopian tube where one loving and perfect sperm penetrates my loving and perfect egg. Delighted with its fertilization, my newly fertilized egg allows the hairlike fibers that line my fallopian tube to move it along. After a relaxing journey of about a week or so my fertilized egg reaches the fluffy and receptive lining of my uterus and easily burrows into it. All systems are communicating. Now my lining starts to release H.C.G., one of my pregnancy hormones. My H.C.G. says to my corpus luteum, "We're a team now. Please stay alive and continue to release progesterone to sustain me. I need your assistance. I'm the nourisher for now." My corpus luteum responds, "I'm releasing. I'll sustain you. You can trust me." Now my corpus luteum feels safe and decides to live long enough for my developing placenta to take over the function of providing nutrition for my embryo. I can see that my placenta is growing normally and sufficiently and oxygen and nutrients are being transported to my healthy fetus. My endometrium is maintained. My body is accepting both my half of my fetus' tissue and its fathers half. I am proud of my body and certainly that includes my strong and competent cervix. It remains closed until my healthy baby has reached full term. At that time it will easily efface and dilate. I am pregnant and feel deeply fulfilled. It is easy for me to find balance in my life. All things fall into place as I relax and trust and let go.

The images that I have created for this self-hypnosis and visualization are simply tools for you. If you have a desire to alter this imagery or symbolize it or make it more personalized, feel free to do so. Play with your images. Spend time. Enjoy the process.

Script II: I.V.F.

Use the same self-hypnosis process as in Script I and continue with the following imagery:

IMAGERY II

I sleep well the night before my egg retrieval. My eggs are mature and well shaped. Soon they are exposed to the washed and capacitated sperm which makes them easily able to penetrate the membrane surrounding my eggs. If necessary a single sperm is injected directly into the cytoplasm of my egg. The quality of all my eggs and the sperm is excellent. All of my eggs fertilize and we have perfect pre-embryos. Again I sleep well the night before my implantation procedure. I am well rested. The embryos are gently transferred to my uterus. The lining of my uterus is a perfect endometrial nest and I see one (or two if you choose) embryo burrow its way into my fluffy receptive lining and attach. I have conceived. I am now pregnant. All systems are communicating. Now my lining starts to release H.C.G., one of my pregnancy hormones. My H.C.G. says to my corpus luteum, "We're a team now. Please stay alive and continue to release progesterone to sustain me. I need your assistance. I'm the nourisher for now." My corpus luteum responds, "I'm releasing. I'll sustain you. You can trust me." Now my corpus luteum feels safe and decides to live long enough for my developing placenta to take over the function of providing nutrition for my embryo. I can see that my placenta is growing normally and sufficiently and oxygen and nutrients are being transported to my healthy fetus. My endometrium is maintained. My body is accepting both my half of my fetus' tissue and its fathers half. I am proud of my body and that includes my strong and competent cervix. It remains closed until my healthy baby has reached full term. At that time, it will easily efface and dilate. I am pregnant and feel deeply fulfilled. It is easy for me to find a balance in my life. All things fall into place as I relax and trust and let go.

Chapter Five

Food: Another Path to Fertility

As you can see, this book is about how to stimulate your own inner fertility potential. You are learning how to deactivate the responses that lead to stress, physical illness and infertility and how to create new pathways that lead to creativity, creation and the life force. Let's continue with the body, the mind, and your hormones.

Physical health is of the utmost importance for conditioning and toning both the male and the female reproductive system.

A naturally balanced diet enhances mind/body, sexual fulfillment and reproductive flow.

Due to improper diet there is often a block of life energy along the primary reproductive channel through fat and mucous accumulation (this information is for men and women).

This can easily be corrected by eliminating over 3 months

*Marijuana and all other non-prescription drugs, including alcohol.

Butter, milk, cheese, eggs.

Meat.

---

* Women are born with a lifetime quota of eggs and use of drugs can damage all of the eggs you have for your lifetime. A man produces a new sperm supply approximately every 100 days.

Sugar—Soft Drinks

Oily—greasy and fried foods

Forget it you may say I'd rather sell my house and spend the money on technology to get us pregnant. This is too much work. Having a baby should be easy and fun.

I understand. I used to think that also. I remember one day when I was 23 and I was wheeling my first baby in his carriage in New York City I saw a woman much older than I walking a walk that implied energy, vitality, life force, litheness. We had the same long, lean body build and hers seemed to go with her, mine felt like I was dragging it along. I envied her. I felt deeply sad and wished for her energy. I was nursing my baby, eating red, white, and brown meat and candies and rhubarb pie and smoking. Formal exercise was unheard of.

Over the years I stopped smoking, stopped eating meat, had 2 more babies, started swimming—and became more and more energized and happy and fulfilled. I can dance till dawn with no problem now that my main drink is green tea, an occasional red wine or champagne. No I don't feel deprived I love the food I eat and remember that woman and today decades later I can walk as she did full of vitality and the life force.

So is it worth changing your eating habits for mental clarity, energy, serenity and joy and a beautiful healthy baby boy or girl. It may seem a difficult choice if you plan to do it overnight. Make your goals easier to meet than not to meet. Decide to do it gradually over a 12 week period. Rather than thinking that you are depriving yourself, realize that you are giving yourself a gift of energy and time. *Improving your diet increases your chances of the effectiveness of your fertility procedures.*

More than 2 million American couples have fertility problems. Between 1965 and 1982 infertility increased from 4% to 10%. Couples are considered infertile if they try to conceive for 1 year without success. Annually billions of pounds of pesticides and industrial compounds that imitate estrogen and/or inhibit testosterone are sprayed on crops and yards and released into waterways. Most of these pollutants accumulate in the fat of beef, fish and other animals.

Male Infertility Factors:
1.   Faulty Semen.

An average ejaculation of 2—3 cubic centimeters of semen contains up to 200—400 million sperms. When the sperm count goes below 50 million per cc there is difficulty with fertilization.

At 25 million there is usually a diagnosis of infertility with a possibility of conception. At 5—10 million sperm conception is difficult.

There can be sufficient number of sperm but they can be either immature or too weak to make it through the female reproductive tract. At least 60% of a sufficient sperm cell count must be mature and be motile.

When there is no apparent reason (like injury, inflammation, or mumps) for the inability to produce an adequate number of quality sperm there is often an underlying dietary, drug and/or psychodynamic cause.

2.   Varicocele and varicose veins in the scrotum this can also cause decreased sperm counts and diminished motility.

Dietary extremes can also cause this disorder.

3.   Duct Blockage.

A blockage in the conveyance between the testes and the penis can be caused by a vasectomy on infection or again dietary causes.

Dietary Treatment:

1. Faulty Semen: Decrease or eliminate drugs, coffee soft drinks, sugar, fruit, fruit juice, chocolate, spices, alcohol, chemical toxins.
2. Varicocele:. Decrease and move toward eliminating cheese, sugar, drugs, soft drinks, coffee, fruit and juices.
3. Duct Blockage. Decrease and move toward eliminating dairy products, fatty oily, greasy foods, animal fats and proteins, sugar.

Cleansing diet—12 week plan—begin to eat fish (fresh farmed), all grains (except wheat), fresh vegetables juices and fresh vegetables, miso soup, soy milk, soy cheese, Bancha tea, green tea, Raja tea (See Nutrition Wheel). To make it simple think in terms of adding healthy foods. Eat healthy foods first and if you have room eat the unhealthy. You'll eventually be enough in balance that you won't even want the unhealthy.

Female Infertility Factors.

Failure to Ovulate.

a) A malfunction in the reproduction of normal egg cells is responsible for about 20% of female infertility.
b) The inability to produce an egg cell (called anovulation) is often accompanied by an hormonal imbalance.

This can be caused by a premature aging of the ovaries or a thickening of the surface of the ovary. In the former instance no eggs remain to mature in the latter ovulation occurs infrequently.

Dietary causes: Excessive intake of fatty animal foods (eggs, cheese, meat, cream). Greasy, high fat foods.

Too much or too little bodily fat. Cleansing diet same as for male (See nutrition wheel). 12 week plan—fish, all grains (except wheat), fresh vegetable juices daily carrot, celery, parsley, beet, ginger, fresh lemon, (this combination actually taste very good) fresh cooked vegetables, miso soup, soy

FOOD: ANOTHER PATH TO FERTILITY   57

milk, soy cheese Bancha tea, Kukicha tea, green tea, Raja cup (tastes like coffee) excellent antioxidant. To order Raja Cup 1–800–255–8332.

Endometriosis.

Portions of the lining of the uterus break away and start growing in other part of the pelvis e.g. the fallopian tubes or ovaries. This tissue can block the reproductive pathways and can cause an hormonal imbalance.

Dietary Causes: All animal products especially fatty, oily and greasy foods, pizza, hamburgers, fried chicken, French fries, sugar, sweets, alcohol and drugs.

Don't worry, shortly we'll get to what you can eat and enjoy.

Fallopian Tube Blockage.

Very common and may result from endometriosis or pelvic inflammations often there is no apparent cause.

Dietary Causes: Even with a severe infection the kinds of food we eat can determine whether or not exposure to a bacteria can cause sterility. Overindulgence of foods rich in fat, protein and salt are unhealthy.

Hostile or Toxic Chemical Mucus.

Toxic mucus can kill any sperm cells with which the mucus has contact. This is the cause of about 10% of infertility in women.

Dietary causes: Overconsumption of greasy, oily foods, animal fats and dairy.

Abortion.

You can greatly enhance your chances of conception through integrating our mind/body program with your treatment plan. Our research is not complete. Anecdotally we have excellent results in enhancing the success of your other fertility treatments.

Standard Healing Diet

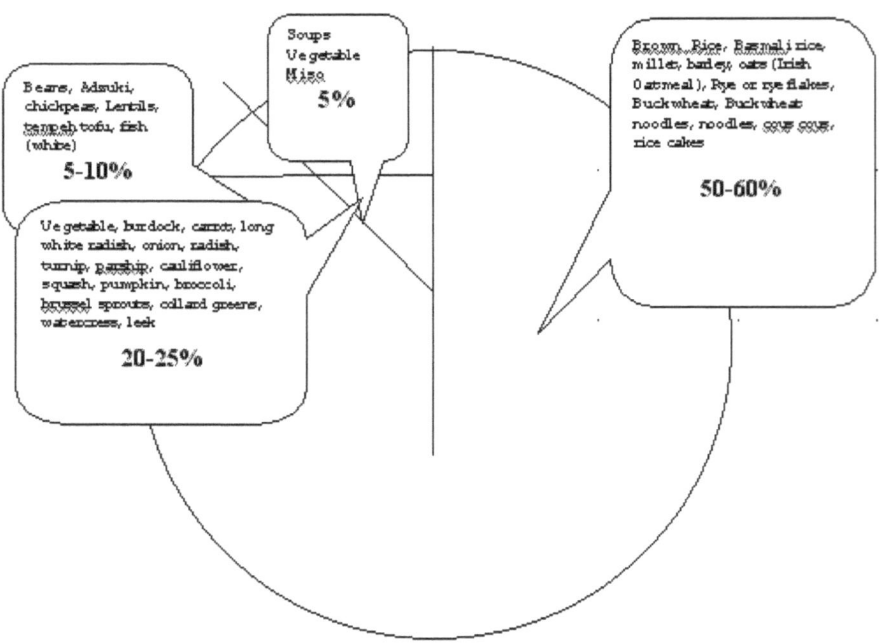

Other vegetables and beans may be eaten. However these are the recommended.

If you have never been to a health food store you might try one if it is available to you. It is quite an adventure. Decide to spend some time reading labels and checking things out. Some of the same products may be available less expensively in your own local market.

Miso Soup is available in paste form in a plastic container and is usually refrigerated. It is great as a quick fix. Just take a heaping tsp. or more and mix in a cup of the hot water and sip as a beverage (get white or yellow miso, its milder).

Boil water with grated ginger, let cool and add fresh lemon and sip throughout the day to cleanse your body and rid it of toxins. It is also satisfying to the digestive system and has a fresh taste.

Well we have now looked at many of the infertility factors from a dietary point of view. These same factors also have a psychological component.

Chapter Six

The Mind/Body As System

To maintain the health and vitality of the reproductive system the entire body needs to be energized. Sexual energy can become manifest through creative, mental and spiritual tonification.

It is a good idea to rest your sexual energies for one to two lunar cycles. This increases the potency of the sperm and diminishes any allergy to the sperm. During this lunar resting cycle become aware of the feelings that emerge having to do with many different aspects of your life. Allow yourself to feel the feelings and to express your feelings, through writing them, sharing them with your partner or with some other person or group. Evidence shows that repression of feelings versus expression is unhealthy for the immune system, thus effecting your reproductive system as well. Confiding improves health.

During this lunar resting cycle it is important to go to sleep between 9 and 10:30 p.m. and to rise after 8 hours of rest. It is also important to sleep separate from your spouse in another room at least once a week. At this time other feelings are given space and time to emerge through the dream cycle. Even if you don't remember your dreams. Dreaming the dream can be healing.[*]

[*] When you get pregnant see Creative Childbirth with Hypnosis by Michelle Leclaire O'Neill, Ph.D., RN for the chapter on working the dream

When you resume sexual activity it is a good idea to wait until ovulation to do so. Decide to go away together during the 1st ovulation to a quiet place in nature where there are no interruptions like phones and computers and TVs. Try to spend 24 hours together alone just being with each other without any pressures of this time bound world. Leave your watches at home and unplug the clocks. Listen to the music of nature and choose a book that will enhance your well being.

Reproductive debility can and does lead couples to reproductive technology. Reproductive technology can detract from romance and sexual vitality and can cause disharmony. Therefore, reproductive system disorders can exacerbate difficulties in relationships, feelings of rejection sexual exhaustion, fear, decrease in confidence and depression.

Exercises.

In order to conceive, a safe environment must be created.

As you go through the following questions there are three rules.

1. Write the first thing that comes to your mind.
2. Keep no secrets from yourself.
3. Have a safe place to keep your writing so that no one can read it unless you want them to do so. (That may mean renting a safe box at a bank or buying a box for home or your car. Decide to do whatever it takes so that your can be free to explore your thoughts and resultant feelings. Take your time and also choose a safe environment for yourself (the beach, home, a restaurant, café, the woods) as you answer the following questions:

Parent I

1.   Why would a baby want to be born into your household?

....

....

....

....

....

....

....

....

....

....

....

....

....

....

Parent II

1.   Why would a baby want to be born into your household?

....

....

....

....

....

....

....

....

....

....

....

....

....

....

Parent I
2.   Why wouldn't a baby want to be born into your household?

....

....

....

....

....

....

....

....

....

....

....

....

....

....

Parent II

2.   Why wouldn't a baby want to be born into your household?

....

....

....

....

....

....

....

....

....

....

....

....

....

....

Parent I

3.   What is predictable about your relationship with your spouse?

....

....

....

....

....

....

....

....

....

....

....

....

....

....

Parent II

3.   What is predictable about your relationship with your spouse?

....

....

....

....

....

....

....

....

....

....

....

....

....

....

....

Parent I

4.   What is not predictable?

....

....

....

....

....

....

....

....

....

....

....

....

....

....

Parent II

4.   What is not predictable?

....

....

....

....

....

....

....

....

....

....

....

....

....

....

Parent I
5.   What do you trust about your spouse?

....

....

....

....

....

....

....

....

....

....

....

....

....

....

Parent II

5.   What do you trust about your spouse?

....

....

....

....

....

....

....

....

....

....

....

....

....

....

Parent I

6.   What don't you trust?

....

....

....

....

....

....

....

....

....

....

....

....

....

....

Parent II

6.   What don't you trust?

....

....

....

....

....

....

....

....

....

....

....

....

....

....

....

Parent I

7.   What about your relationship allows you to feel safe?

....

....

....

....

....

....

....

....

....

....

....

....

....

....

Parent II

7.   What about your relationship allows you to feel safe?

....

....

....

....

....

....

....

....

....

....

....

....

....

....

Parent I

8.   Is there anything in your relationship that gives rise to feelings of not being safe?

....

....

....

....

....

....

....

....

....

....

....

....

....

Parent II

8.   Is there anything in your relationship that gives rise to feelings of not being safe?

....

....

....

....

....

....

....

....

....

....

....

....

....

Parent I

9.   What are fears that you had as a child that you don't have today?

....

....

....

....

....

....

....

....

....

....

....

....

....

....

Parent II

9.   What are fears that you had as a child that you don't have today?

....

....

....

....

....

....

....

....

....

....

....

....

....

....

Parent I

10.   What are fears that you had as an adolescent that you don't have today?

....

....

....

....

....

....

....

....

....

....

....

....

....

....

Parent II

10.   What are fears that you had as an adolescent that you don't have today?

....

....

....

....

....

....

....

....

....

....

....

....

....

....

Parent I

11.   What are fears that you may have had in the past that continue into the present?

....

....

....

....

....

....

....

....

....

....

....

....

....

Parent II

11.   What are fears that you may have had in the past that continue into the present?

....

....

....

....

....

....

....

....

....

....

....

....

....

....

Parent I

12.   What are your fears concerning marriage, conception, pregnancy, birth, breastfeeding and parenting?

....

....

....

....

....

....

....

....

....

....

....

....

....

....

Parent II

12.   What are your fears concerning marriage, conception, pregnancy, birth, breastfeeding and parenting?

....

....

....

....

....

....

....

....

....

....

....

....

....

....

Parent I

13.   What do you like about your present relationship with your spouse?

....

....

....

....

....

....

....

....

....

....

....

....

....

Parent II

13.   What do you like about your present relationship with your spouse?

....

....

....

....

....

....

....

....

....

....

....

....

....

....

Parent I

14.   How do you perceive *pregnancy* altering your relationships?

....

....

....

....

....

....

....

....

....

....

....

....

....

....

Parent II

14.   How do you perceive *pregnancy* altering your relationships?

....

....

....

....

....

....

....

....

....

....

....

....

....

....

....

Parent I

15.   How do you perceive *having* a *child* and being a parent would alter your relationship?

....

....

....

....

....

....

....

....

....

....

....

....

....

....

Parent II

15.   How do you perceive *having* a *child* and being a parent would alter your relationship?

....

....

....

....

....

....

....

....

....

....

....

....

....

Parent I

16.   What would you like about being a parent?

....

....

....

....

....

....

....

....

....

....

....

....

....

....

Parent II

16.   What would you like about being a parent?

....

....

....

....

....

....

....

....

....

....

....

....

....

....

....

Parent I
17.   What do you think you wouldn't like?

....

....

....

....

....

....

....

....

....

....

....

....

....

....

Parent II

17.   What do you think you wouldn't like?

....

....

....

....

....

....

....

....

....

....

....

....

....

....

Parent I

18.   Are your feelings about pregnancy, birth and parenting your own or have they been imposed upon you by your own parents or others? Explain in writing to yourself.

....

....

....

....

....

....

....

....

....

....

....

....

....

....

Parent II

18.   Are your feelings about pregnancy, birth and parenting your own or have they been imposed upon you by your own parents or others? Explain in writing to yourself.

....

....

....

....

....

....

....

....

....

....

....

....

....

....

Parent I

19.   What thoughts and feelings do you want to keep around pregnancy, birth, and parenting?

....

....

....

....

....

....

....

....

....

....

....

....

....

....

Parent II

19.   What thoughts and feelings do you want to keep around pregnancy, birth, and parenting?

....

....

....

....

....

....

....

....

....

....

....

....

....

....

Parent I
20.   What thoughts and feelings do you want to let go?

....

....

....

....

....

....

....

....

....

....

....

....

....

....

Parent II

20.   What thoughts and feelings do you want to let go?

....

....

....

....

....

....

....

....

....

....

....

....

....

....

Before letting go of any problems, it is important to name them; to acknowledge them, to discuss them with a safe, non-judgmental person to arrive at the underlying thoughts and attitudes behind the problem and the pursuant feelings. We already explained unhealthy thinking and learned how to reframe it so that problems could be viewed as a signal for change not as a sign of weakness and passivity helplessness and hopelessness.

I have found both through my own analysis and meditation and dreams as well as through work with patients that letting go is a process not a cathartic event. We may let go of a thought/feeling today only to have it reemerge tomorrow. Since we have done the work today it becomes easier tomorrow and easier still the next day and the next to let go. And then there may come a day when some demon of which we have certainly rid ourselves vehemently rears his ugly and perhaps frightening head and we must redecide to return to the path of wellness and begin our work anew. However, this time with the confidence of "I have done this before. It is horrific to have it reenter my being and I can deal with it." I have found that all of the tools and techniques of this program are simple ways of moving forward on the path of mind/body/spirit healing.

Chapter Seven

Psychobiology of Emotions/Immune System/Reproduction

In order for the trophoblast to survive, the mothers immune system needs to be able to produce certain antibodies.

When the antibody binds with the trophoblast antigen then the growth and cell division necessary for the pregnancy to flourish takes place. If this does not happen and the trophoblast dies then additional adverse immune responses occur which can lead to recurrent pregnancy losses.

It is suggested that an immunological evaluation be done for all couples following their second loss. There are physiological pathways that connect the brain to the immune system which in turn may effect the maternal antibody binding to the necessary paternal lymphocytes which is necessary for healthy growth and development of the trophoblast and its further development into a healthy embryo and viable fetus.

Let us look for a moment at the Hypothalamus-Pituitary-Adrenal Axis which responds to stress and emotions:

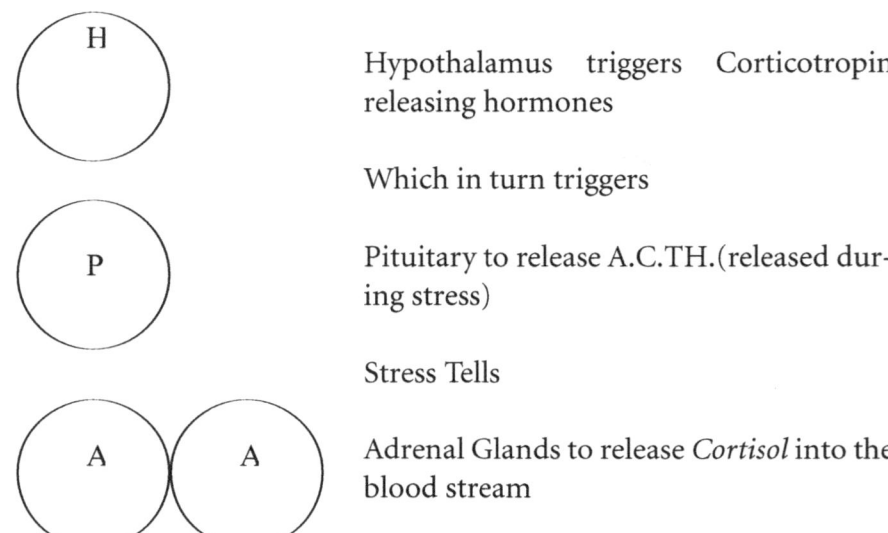

Hypothalamus triggers Corticotropin releasing hormones

Which in turn triggers

Pituitary to release A.C.TH.(released during stress)

Stress Tells

Adrenal Glands to release *Cortisol* into the blood stream

Too much cortisol is unhealthy and persistent stress can break down the cortisol regulating system. Too much cortisol can cause apoptosis or cell suicide.

It appears that people with negative expectations do something detrimental to the physiology of their bodies. Persistent negative expectations can become feelings of hopelessness and helplessness, this leading to depression.

Depression is associated with decreased antibody response and decreased antibody response as we spoke of above may cause recurrent pregnancy losses'.

The brain and the psyche and the body are connected. The stress hormone Cortisol in excess suppresses digestion and reproduction. Oftentimes couples trying to become pregnant move in the direction of negative expectations and hopelessness and lack of control. Therefore it is imperative to prevent this negative cycle.

How to Prevent this Negative Cycle

1. Take back control—i.e. do as much as you can yourselves (work exercises in book)
2. Begin a Nutrition Plan
3. Exercise
4. Change your thinking from unhealthy to healthy
5. Establish realistic goals
6. Use your Relaxation tools
    a. Hypnosis—can change physiology (Hypno Fertility tape*)
    b. Imagery—also can change physiology and increase positive expectations and a sense of control (Healing tape*)
    c. Meditation—returns body to optimal health
    d. Confiding—Improves general health and the immune system
7. Maintain Fertile Relationships
8. Social Support
9. Play

---

* For ordering information - See back of book

Chapter Eight

Fertile Relationships

Fertile relationships have a capacity for adaptation by both parties.

The work that each person does in the relationship may be fun or a drag, a joy, a drudge. However it is most important that one feels fulfilled by his or her work and if this is not so, imagine what you can do to make it so? A fertile relationship begins with a person's own creativity. Each person must have a way of expressing his/her own uniqueness and have a feeling of accomplishment. A fertile environment must be created which can be as simple as a quiet place to sleep and to dine without TV, sufficient rest and exercise on a regular basis, time alone together.

Fertility is not about winning- it is about letting go and letting yourself and the other person feel empowered and enriched. It is also asking for what you want and not feeling guilty when you get what you want. Learn to accept yes gently and graciously. If you must say no and receive a no also do that gently and graciously. Acknowledge your own limitations and your partner's and work within that frame. Be gentle with yourself and others

How to move towards fertile relationships.

1.   Take quiet time each day—minimum 1/2 hour for yourself and respect your partner's quiet time. Do whatever you feel like doing without any goals. Therefore, this does not mean clean the refrigerator, clean off your desk, attack a pile of bills.

It does mean:

Unplug the phone and stare at the ceiling
Listen to music
Read
Take a bath
Give yourself a massage
Watch a sunrise or sunset
Play an instrument
Take a stroll
Blow bubbles
Paint or draw or sketch
Meditate
Watch the clouds or the waves
Listen to the breeze or the birds

Make up your list and show it to each other. It can be a good time to learn about each other needs and desires.

Parent I
Things I would like to do for myself in my quiet time alone.

....

....

....

....

....

....

....

....

....

....

....

....

....

....

Parent II
Things I would like to do for myself in my quiet time alone.

....

....

....

....

....

....

....

....

....

....

....

....

....

....

2.   Identify your social support system—From whom and how do you receive it (phone, family, classes, meetings, groups, church, synagogue, temple) Make a list of where you get your social support. Is this fulfilling to you? What would you like to delete and what would you like to add? Social support can greatly add to a fertile life and to cultivating fertile relationships.

Move toward people not away from them. The right people in your life can enhance your relationship, to yourself, to your spouse and to your own reproductivity.

3.   Exercise

Exercise is a significant factor in dealing positively with emotions and as we have learned emotions affect our reproductive system. To move is to be alive. Exercise provides a physiological outlet for stress. It gives one a sense of taking charge of creating some order and power over ones life. It also decreases depression and enhances feelings of well-being. Exercise is a natural mood elevator. It's a dietless form of weight control and a sedative without the negative side effects. Its therapy without payment and a face lift without the surgery.

It is one of the best gifts you can give to yourself. Its as simple as walking out your front door and going around the block. It's as simple as taking the stairs instead of the elevator. It's as simple as…. (you can fill in the blank to suit your own needs)

Chapter Nine

Twelve Week Health Plan

Development of your health plan is the framework of your 12 week fertility program.

Your life's activities have been artificially divided into six categories:

1. Play
2. Exercise
3. Social Support
4. Nutrition
5. Creative healing, which includes meditation, hypnosis (Hypno-Fertility), Imagery, Visualization, Dreamwork, therapeutic touch, acupuncture and massage.

Would you please now take the time to identify which is most important to your overall wellbeing. Take time to contemplate this 2 or 3 days and then develop and write out your plan. This is a guide to let you know the direction you are going and the pace you are setting for yourself. Write the plan in pencil. Make each goal a baby step i.e. make the goal easier to meet then not to meet.

It is important for you to know that you are always free to alter your plan: the plan is simply the framework upon which you can expand.

Start slowly, the blackout spaces are there for you to add a new step gradually. Continue to be gentle with yourself. Take your time "It takes as long as it takes."

	Week 1	Week 2/3	Week 4/5	Week 6/7	Week 8	Week 9	Week 10/11	Week 12
Creative Healing Meditation Hypnosis	I will focus on my breath with my eyes closed for 5 minutes	Continue week 1 + I'll listen to Hypnofertility tape (2x)	No change	I'll use a MANTRA PACEM for 10 min 2x will continue hypnofertility tape	No change	Increase meditation to 10 min 3x; and continue hypnofertilit y 2x week	Meditation 10 min 3x; Hypnofertility tape 3x	No change
Social Support		Go to nature with partner and sit on beach and listen to surf x1 for 15 min	Continue beach, go to concert or theatre with partner x1	No change	Continue as before — plan a weekend trip for week 12	Continue as before — have dinner with another couple-out group x1 (50min)	Go out with girlfriends shopping, Romantic weekend away	Continue as before plus weekend away
Exercise			Walk outside for 10 min 1x this week	Do 5 min of stretching x1 and walk outside 10 min x2	No change	5 min stretch x2 walk outside 20 min x2	No change	5 min stretch x3 walk outside 20 min x3
Play				Turn phone off; read for 20 min(not work related)	Continue as before— take bubble baths with candles (no phone)	Continue as before - turn on Reggae music and dance	No change	Continue as before plus get facial
Nutrition					Take prenatal vitamins daily	Eliminate alcohol and carbonated drinks	Continue as before and research a good nutrition book	Continue as before Buy book and read it and/or follow instructions on Sample plan Nutrition

	Week 1	Week 2/3	Week 4/5	Week 6/7	Week 8	Week 9	Week 10/11	Week 12
Creative Healing Meditation Hypnosis								
Social Support	▒							
Exercise	▒	▒						
Play	▒	▒	▒					
Nutrition	▒	▒	▒	▒				

	Week 1	Week 2/3	Week 4/5	Week 6/7	Week 8	Week 9	Week 10/11	Week 12
Creative Healing Meditation Hypnosis								
Social Support								
Exercise								
Play								
Nutrition								

	Week 1	Week 2/3	Week 4/5	Week 6/7	Week 8	Week 9	Week 10/11	Week 12
Creative Healing Meditation Hypnosis								
Social Support								
Exercise								
Play								
Nutrition								

	Week 1	Week 2/3	Week 4/5	Week 6/7	Week 8	Week 9	Week 10/11	Week 12
Creative Healing Meditation Hypnosis								
Social Support								
Exercise								
Play								
Nutrition								

	Week 1	Week 2/3	Week 4/5	Week 6/7	Week 8	Week 9	Week 10/11	Week 12
Creative Healing Meditation Hypnosis								
Social Support	▒							
Exercise	▒	▒						
Play	▒	▒	▒					
Nutrition	▒	▒	▒	▒				

Short Term Goals

1.   Decide to move in the direction of healthy foods and away from animal products.

2.   Formulate a weekly realistic goal around your eating—do a 3 month plan.

3.   Women—Begin taking prenatal vitamins.

4.   Men—Begin taking a well-rounded vitamin/mineral formula daily.

5.   Meet with spouse 15 minutes each week to discuss eating plan and feelings about it.

6.   Schedule play into your life, separately and together each week. Play enhances the immune and reproductive system

Definition of Play—Play is having fun and is not goal oriented.

Week 1	Week 2	Week 3	Week 4	Week 5	Week 6	Week 7	Week 8	Week 9	Week 10	Week 11	Week 12
Drink Miso Soup at Break-fast	Continue Miso; find store that makes fresh vegetable juice drink 3x this week	Drink H_2O, lemon, ginger through out the day	Continue H_2O lemon vegetable juice this week	No animal products this week; drink 4 on Monday eat whole grains	No animal products this week; Mon and Thurs continue extra grains	Eat 3 new vegetables this week	No animal products 3 days this week; add beans to diet	Find health food store	Drink 6 vegetable juices this week; buy electric rice & vegetable steamer	Eat 2 natural foods 4 days this week choose from standard healing diet	Eat standard healing diet 5 days this week

	Week 1
	Week 2
	Week 3
	Week 4
	Week 5
	Week 6
	Week 7
	Week 8
	Week 9
	Week 10
	Week 11
	Week 12

	Week 1	Week 2	Week 3	Week 4	Week 5	Week 6	Week 7	Week 8	Week 9	Week 10	Week 11	Week 12

Congratulations! You have completed the reading of this book. Now go back to page 37 and follow the instructions for doing the exercises. Being involved in your own treatment in this way decreases your anxiety and enhances your chances of success. Be a healing partner with *yourself.*
Take your time and enjoy the work that you are doing.
You may now begin to write in your fertility journal on Page 152, whenever you are ready.

Chapter Ten

Your Fertility Journal

I once thought that if I worked hard at something and prepared I would succeed. In the past that has been true. Why isn't that so now?

Earthly things so fade, decay,
Constant to us not one day;
Suddenly they pass away,
And we cannot make them stay.

Elizabeth Stuart

Thoughts on Acceptance:

....

....

....

....

It has been a long time since we decided to get pregnant. I look at other pregnant woman with envy. Sometimes I can't even look at them.

"Forgive me if I am incapable of weeping, of simple human weeping, but instead keep singing and running..."

Vladimir Nabokov

Thoughts on Forgiveness:

....

....

....

....

....

....

I used to be so concerned about watching my weight and having a flat belly. Now all I want is a grand pregnant abdomen. I don't even care about gaining weight. I want to be pregnant.

O dream of joy! is this indeed
the lighthouse top I see?
Is this the hill? is this the kirk?
Is this mine own Countree?

Samuel Taylor Coleridge

Thoughts on Hope

....

....

....

....

....

....

I'm tired of all of this. I feel as though I have no control and am on an hormonal roller coaster. I want to be more in touch with my body.

Where are the songs of spring? Ay, where are they?

John Keats

My feelings about my non-pregnant body:

....

....

....

....

....

....

❀ ☀ ❅

I have been thinking about starting a barrage of tests and perhaps medications and invasive procedures. It seems easier that way. I'm tired. Let technology do it.

—*Then on the shore*
Of the wide world I stand alone, and think.

John Keats

Thoughts on medications and their side effects:

....

....

....

....

....

....

I need a definitive diagnosis before I can proceed. I don't believe in the diagnosis unexplained infertility. Perhaps the answer lies deep within my psyche or the psyche of our marriage.

In a drear-nighted December,
  Too happy happy brook,
Thy bubblings ne'er remember
  Apollo's summer look;

John Keats

Thoughts about exploring the unknown:

....

....

....

....

....

....

....

❀ ☀ ❆

I need to take charge of my own fertility. Perhaps its as simple as my diet or exercising too much or too little.

Blow, bugle, blow set the wild echoes flying.

Alfred Tennyson

My unedited thoughts about my lifestyle:

....

....

....

....

....

....

❀ ☼ ❊

All we think about and talk about is getting pregnant. I wish I could focus on other things but its very difficult. I feel sad and angry and tired.

The camel has a single hump;
the dromedary, two;
Or else the other way around.
I'm never sure are you?

Ogden Nash

Things that bring me joy.

....

....

....

....

....

....

❋ ◉ ✢

I've been too upset. Why would a baby want to grow in my uterus? I need to invite the soul of my baby into my body.

My boreal lights leap upward,
Forthright my planets roll,
And still the man-child is not born,
The summit of the whole.

Ralph Waldo Emerson

Letter and invitation to my baby:

....

....

....

....

....

....

I'm buying into this fertility technology the way I bought brought into having a vogue body. Today I shall *STOP* and draw up a plan around nutrition and a fertility diet.

Between the moon and the sun
There's time to pluck a tune upon the harp.

Dylan Thomas

Thoughts on Hope

....

....

....

....

....

....

It is difficult for me to take the time to do this naturally. I feel that time is running out. I want to be in control.

Well, what shall I do today?
Shall I spend the day in the hay?
Shall I cover my head with the sheets,
Or go downstairs and eat?

Ogden Nash

Thoughts on Letting Go.

....

....

....

....

....

....

I either exercise too much or too little. I need to learn moderation.

Shall I walk a mile or run?
Shall I skip in the sand to have fun?
Shall I climb a mountain high
Or aerobically reach for the sky?

Michelle Leclaire

Today I'll draw up a realistic exercise plan:

....

....

....

....

....

....

Life has become very serious. I often forget how to have fun. Play is rarely a part of my life.

I never take the time to play
Or sit and dream a day away
I only chart my menstual trends
Beginning, middle, and over again.

Michelle Leclaire

Today I shall make a play list of 10 things I can do alone and 10 things I'd like to do together:

....

....

....

....

....

....

I have lost sight of my purpose in life. It seems that my passion is gone. My only purpose is to conceive.

The summer voice so warm from fruit
That clustered round her shoulders…

Dylan Thomas

Other areas I can focus on that allow me to feel fertile:

....

....

....

....

....

....

My thinking is no longer creative and free. I am often obsessed by infertile thoughts.

Sperm and eggs my thoughts are of
Whatever happened to our love.
at 5:09 I ovulate
Come home my dear please don't be late

Michelle Leclaire

Today I shall write out my infertile thoughts and change them to healthier more fertile thinking:

Unhealthy Infertile thoughts   Healthy Rational thoughts

_____   _____
_____   _____
_____   _____
_____   _____
_____   _____
_____   _____

It remains difficult for me to think clearly at times. I continue to compulsively think about having a baby. Today I shall begin a program of emptying my mind of all thoughts. No T.V., no phone, no radio, no tapes, no music. I'll repeat aloud to myself a mantra—*PACEM*. I'll say it more and more softly until it is inaudible even to me. I shall focus only on the word pacem for 20 minutes.

Than smoke and mist who better could appraise
The kindred spirit of an inner haze.

Robert Frost

The best time and place for me to regularly still my mind is:

I shall begin doing this on _____

date

I shall do this_____

how many times a week

....

....

....

....

....

❀ ☀ ❉

It would be nice if I could meet other women who are dealing with similar issues. This is an isolating experience. I don't really want to talk about fertility or infertility but I do want to relate in some way.

"Anne! or whoever you are, dear…
Or not dear;
Well…Zoe! Nadjejdu! Jane!
Look! I'm strolling here
Lined with gold like the skies!
English spoken?—Spanish?
Batignolle.

Tristan Corbiere

Creative ways of meeting and sharing with other women:

1. _____

2. _____

3. _____

4. _____

5. _____

6. _____

Epilogue

What is Life?
It is a shooting star across a midnight sky
It is the fleeting scent of orange blossom and lilac
It is the shadow that runs across the hill
It is the Pink moment that glows upon the mountain and slips
till dawn beneath the valley floor

Congratulations on completing the work in this book. Please continue your 12-week plan.

"It works if you work it"

Order Form

Fertility in 12 Weeks — —

Fertility Tape (Hypnofertility) — $9.95

Fertility CD (Hypnofertility) — 10.95

Healing Tape — 9.95

Creative Childbirth:

The Complete Leclaire Hypnobirthing Method — 12.95

Leclaire Pregnancy Workbook — 6.95

The Pregnancy Diary

(a lovely daily journal and keepsake a must for every couple)

Hypnobirthing Pregnancy Tape or CD	9.95 Tape	10.95 CD
Hypnobirthing Labor Tape or CD	9.95 Tape	10.95 CD
Music tape or CD—Bach for	9.95 Tape	10.95 CD
Babies and their Mothers		

Scientifically tested, excellent for ADD & ADHD

The Umbilical Code Paper — 1.95

  (Is the mother growing a body/brain or is she also creating the mind of her child)

We ship Priority Mail in 24-48 hours—add $4.25 for shipping and handling for 1 to 5 items and add $4.00 for over 5 items

Subtotal: _____.___
CA Tax (8.25%): _____.___
Shipping & Handling: _____.___
TOTAL DUE: _____.___

Send check or money order only payable to:
Michelle O'Neill, Ph.D., R.N.
P.O. Box 1086
Pacific Palisades, CA 90272
Phone 310–454–0920
Email: birthing@gte.net
Web site: http://www.hypnobirthing.ws
We accept Credit Cards